# ESSENTIAL OILS FOR SLEEP

Safe And Natural Essential Oils For Insomnia

Tonny M Ford, RN, BSN, PHN.

© 2015

# *Essential*
# *Oils*
## *For Sleep*

## SAFE AND NATURAL ESSENTIAL
## OILS FOR INSOMNIA

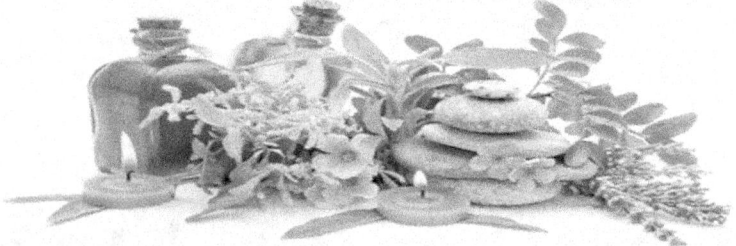

TONNY M FORD, RN, BSN, PHN
## essentialoilRN.net

# Introduction

I want to thank you and congratulate you for purchasing the book, *"Essential Oils for Sleep: Safe and Natural essential oils for insomnia"*.

This book contains proven steps and strategies on how to use different kinds of essential oils to benefit from these, especially in terms of getting better sleep.

It is very important that you get sufficient rest every night, but this is something that not all people have the ability to do quite easily. This book contains information on why you are losing sleep and how you can solve the dilemma by learning what essential oils to use and how. You would also learn about how you can use the essential oils to lift your spirits, manage your mood, relax, and ultimately, get some quality sleep.

Thanks again for purchasing this book. I hope you enjoy it!

# Disclaimer

This document is geared towards providing exact and reliable information in regards to the topic and issue covered. The publication is sold with the idea that the publisher is not required to render accounting, officially permitted, or otherwise, qualified services. If advice is necessary, legal or professional, a practiced individual in the profession should be ordered.

- From a Declaration of Principles which was accepted and approved equally by a Committee of the American Bar Association and a Committee of Publishers and Associations.

In no way is it legal to reproduce, duplicate, or transmit any part of this document in either electronic means or in printed format. Recording of this

using essentials oils or anything that can affect your health. Your doctor is the only one who knows the true story of your health and can give your better professional help.

# Bonus Gift!!

**As a way of saying thank you for purchasing our book**, we have included a free 140 page exclusive pdf report on **essential oils guide**. We believe that that the value in this report will enrich your life abundantly. As a subscriber, you will the first to get a new free ebooks before anyone else! If you have any questions, please contact us at support@essentialoilrn.net

## Click here to download your free bonus ebook

http://www.essentialoilrn.net/thank/

# Table of Contents

# Chapter 1

## Essential Oils and Sleep – An Overview

Essential oils are extracted from plants. The oils have the volatile aroma compound of the plants where these were derived. The oils are also called different terms, such as ethereal oils, volatile oils and aetherolea.

The extraction of the oils from the plants is done through various processes, which include solvent extraction, expression, but the most common method is distillation through the use of a steam. These oils do not have any distinct category for culinary, pharmacological and medicinal purposes. Essential oils are popularly used in perfumes, soaps, cosmetics, various household products and flavors of food and drinks.

There are people who believe that essential oils can help cure sicknesses and diseases, since these have been used in ancient times. There are certain countries, which regulate the products with essential oils that are being promoted as alternative treatments to illnesses, including the management of cancer.

There were years when the popularity of the use of essential oils declined due to the unproven medical claims. The interest in these oils was revived in recent decades with the demand of aromatherapy. In this branch of alternative medicine, the oils are diluted in carrier oil. The final product is then used in a variety of ways.

Aromatherapy can help people and animals to feel better, calm the nerves, relieve certain aches and a lot more. This is also popularly used to help people and animals get quality sleep.

Do you have any trouble sleeping? It is important to get sufficient rest no matter how young or old you are. The quality of sleep that you get each day affects your mood and performance. This book will help you uncover the top essential oils that you can use in order to sleep better and give insights about the other uses of these oils. Before tackling the topic, here's an overview about the importance of good sleep.

# Why Sleep is Important

Did you know that in the US alone, about 40 million people suffer from different kinds of sleep disorders? Many of these people do not do anything about the condition and they simply let it pass without getting diagnosed and treated.

The amount of sleep that each individual needs varies depending on a lot of factors. In general, healthy adults need an average of eight hours of sleep each night. There are some people who feel weak when they don't get a minimum of 10 hours of sleep, while others feel energized and could no longer go back to bed after sleeping for six hours or less. It is not true that you no longer need the 8-hour sleep rule when you get older. This is still necessary, but the ability to sleep and stay asleep for six to eight hours each night becomes more difficult. This is where the aromatherapy using essential oils will come in handy.

## What causes sleep problems?

The problem with your sleeping patterns is rooted to various causes, which include the following:

- Physiological problems, including emotional disorders, obesity, brain and nervous system disorders.
- Stress can lead to sleep loss. The sleep problem, in this case, is only temporary and will disappear after you have dealt with what's causing the stress.
- Your lifestyle greatly affects your sleeping pattern. Drinking alcohol and caffeine during the day can lead to difficulty in sleeping at night.
- The biological rhythm of those who work on a shifting schedule is likely to get affected, especially in the beginning, as their bodies try to adjust. This can lead to sleepiness at work and finding it hard to sleep when you get home.
- Your circadian rhythm is affected when you travel to places with different time zones than the place where you are from.
- Your surroundings also affect the quality of your sleep. You have to set up your room according to your preferences when it comes to temperature, lighting, and beddings.

## Proper Ways of Using Essential Oils

Different kinds of essential oils have different properties. It is essential that you read the precautions on how and when to use these. You have to know if the oil is safe to use even when undiluted or if moderate or heavy dilution is necessary. It is also important to understand if the oil is safe for children, pregnant women or people who are suffering from certain illnesses.

The following are the most popular ways of using essential oils.

1. Aromatic application. The scents that are coming from the oils are processed by the same system that deals with people's feelings, memories and thoughts. This is the olfactory bulb and the limbic system. The aroma creates positive effects on one's psychological and physical systems. It is able to affect one's mood. The aroma helps in improving the quality of indoor air. It gives protection against airborne contaminants. A person's immune system responds positively with the scent.

The following techniques are used for the aromatic application of essential oils.

- Direct inhalation. This is done by holding the oil's container a few inches away from your nose. You simply have to inhale the aroma, enjoy the process and wait for the scent to take effect. The simpler way to do this is by dropping a small amount in your hands and cupping your hands over your nose to inhale the aroma. There are certain oils, such as cinnamon and oregano, which you cannot inhale directly without diluting the oils first.
- Indirect inhalation. This is done by adding a drop or two of your chosen oil to a cotton ball and putting this near your bed or under your pillow. You can also apply a few drops on your pillow and beddings so that you can inhale the scent while you are in the room or as you sleep. You can opt to put a small amount of oil in the shirt that you are wearing, in your hair, or the handkerchief that you are using.
- Diffusing. Use the kind of diffuser that utilizes a room or cold temperature or ultrasonic vibrations in spreading the scent of the oil into a room. This way, the molecules of the oil remain in the air for more hours than when you use the kind of diffuser that utilizes heat.
- Natural air deodorizer. Instead of using the commercially available deodorizers that may contain harmful chemicals, you can concoct your own that only has natural ingredients.
- Humidifier. Make sure that you choose the type that is specifically made for essential oils. There are certain kinds with plastic components that can deteriorate over time when you use it for essential oils.

- Fan and vent. Add some drops of oil into a cloth and place this in front of a fan or vent. When the appliances are in use, the scent of the oil will naturally get incorporated with the air.

2. Topical Application. Before you apply any oils directly to the skin, make sure that you aren't sensitive to these. Perform a skin patch to test if you are sensitive to the oils or not. While there are certain oils that are safe to use even when undiluted, diluting the oils does not affect its effectiveness.

The following are among the popular ways of using essential oils topically:

- Massage. This is relaxing and comforting, especially when essential oils are used in the process. In doing massages, make sure that are extra careful when dealing with the spine and sensitive areas of the body. In massaging the legs and arms, move gently from the bottom towards the heart.
- Reflexology. Apply a few drops of the oil over your body's reflex points. You can download and print out an image that describes the reflex points and how to deal with these.
- Personal care. You can add essential oils to the products that you use for your skin regimen. These products include deodorants, lotion for the body and moisturizers for the face.

3. Internal application. Before you consume any kind of essential oils, make sure that these are listed as "generally recognized as safe for internal use" by the FDA. It is important to take note that not all kinds of oils are safe to take internally.

- Cooking. Some of the oils that are popularly used in cooking or baking include rosemary and oregano. Use the oils in moderation.
- Drinking. You can add certain oils to your drinks, such as lemon and peppermint. The oils and liquid will not mix, so only add a little of the oil so that you don't find it hard to consume the drink with the oils floating on top.
- Supplemental. There are readily available supplements with essential oils that help various conditions, such as aiding in the digestion process, boosts energy and immunity. You can also create your own supplement by buying empty veggie capsules and filling these with the essential oils of your choice.

## Using Essential Oils to Sleep Better

It is easier to deal with your sleeping problem if you already know what's causing this. Aside from making the necessary adjustment and changes, it is helpful to find out the essential oils that can help you in this regard.

A small bottle of an essential oil can last a long time, depending on how you use it. You can use the oils in different ways in order to help you get a better sleep. Here are some of the ways to use the essential oils to help calm your nerves and prepare you towards a quality slumber.

1. Bathing

Choose the kind of fragrance that is not overpowering. Different people react to the scents in different ways. It may take some trial and error process before you find the right scents that can help you sleep soundly. You will find it easier to sleep when you bathe before you go to bed. Make sure that the lights in the bathroom are set to dim. You can prefer to use the light that is coming from unscented candles. As you prepare your body to sleep, set a relaxing mood as you bathe. It will help if you are going to play a soothing music.

Refrain from having a hot bath before bed because this can stimulate your nerves. Run a warm bath instead. Add three drops of your chosen essential oil to the water. Soak up for at least 10 minutes before you wash your body using an unscented soap or gel. Make sure that you don't use other scents aside from the aroma that the essential oil contains. Mixing two scents in this case might ruin the purpose of preparing your body to bed. Towel your body dry and apply an unscented talcum powder, which can help you feel fresh even as you sleep.

## 2. Topical application

Before you sleep, you can directly apply a drop of your chosen essential oil to your wrists or temples, the areas in your body with high circulation and steady temperature.

## 3. Breathing the aroma first thing upon waking up

After having a good night's sleep, you might find it hard to wake up because your body still feels sleepy from the essential oils that you have chosen to surround yourself with. In this case, there are other scents of essential oils that will help you wake up feeling refreshed and wide awake. These oils include peppermint and citrus. You simply have to inhale the fragrances as you wake your body up and perform your usual exercises.

Quick Notes about Essential Oils

It is better to buy the oils from a physical store than online if it is your first time to do this. You have to try and smell the scents to find out what you prefer, what makes you feel good and light. You can always purchase the oils online when you already know the scents that appeal to you. This is very important because even if an oil is proven to make a lot of people sleep better, it will not have the same effect on you if you don't like its smell. Buy a pure essential oil because this will last longer and perform better.

Take a lot of care when applying the oils directly on your skin. If you develop any allergies in using the oils, consult a doctor immediately.

# Chapter 2

## Lavender Essential Oil

Lavender is known for its versatility, hence, its moniker as the Swiss Army Knife of essential oils. The oil is derived from the spikes of certain kinds of lavender flowers through the process of distillation. There are two distinguished forms of lavender oil. The first one is the lavender spike oil that comes from an herb known as the Lavandula latifolia. This has a higher concentration than the second type, which is the lavender flower oil that has no color and insoluble in water.

This kind of essential oil is not a pure compound, but a complex mixture of certain phytochemicals. The spike oil was commonly used in oil painting before the introduction of distilled turpentine. The smell of this essential oil is popularly used as a scent for cosmetics and perfumes. There has been a controversy about this essential oil when it was believed to cause pre-pubertal gynecomastia, or the unusual growth of breasts, in pre-adolescent boys.

This is included in the list of the most popular essential oils that are used to obtain better sleep. This has a soothing and relaxing effect and can also alleviate anxiety levels.

Other Uses of Lavender Essential Oil

Aside from promoting sleep, since the smell of lavender is relaxing, you can use this for the following purposes:

1. Sunburn. To relieve the skin from the effects of sunburn, you can directly apply two drops of this oil to the affected area. You can also add eight drops of this oil to one teaspoon of jojoba oil and four drops of peppermint oil. Pour the mixture into your warm bath and soak for at least 10 minutes.

2. Insect bites. You can directly apply a drop of this oil on the affected area to help relieve itching and swelling. You can also use this to prevent bites from insects, such as mosquitoes and midges. These insects hate the smell of lavender. You can splash

lavender hydrosol on your body before going outdoors. You can also pour some oil to a cotton ball, place this in an open container and place it beside the window to prevent small insects from coming inside your house.

3. Keeping the laundry smelling fresh. This is a natural way to get the job done. You simply have to apply several drops to the wool dryer balls and let the oil do its work. This can also help in keeping the moths off your clothes. Hang lavender bags inside the closet. Refresh the bag every once in a while by adding a drop of this oil.

4. Muscle aches. After spending the whole day doing bone-breaking tasks, a soak in a lavender warm bath can help in soothing the pains and aches. To deal with muscle tension, pour several drops of lavender oil in your warm bath, along with Epsom salts.

5. Stronger and thicker eyelashes. Add a drop of this oil to your mascara. The result will help the lashes grow naturally and become stronger.

6. Burns and cuts. A drop of this oil can help in disinfecting cuts and relieve the pain that is caused by burns. Add more drops depending on the severity of the condition. For minor burns, you must first immerse the affected area in running water for at least five minutes before massaging it gently with lavender oil. After the pain is gone, the burns will get healed without obvious scars. For cuts and wounds, the oil works wonders as it soothes the pain, prevent infections and formation of scars. You simply have to apply the oil directly to the affected area after you have cleansed the wound.

7. Acne. You can use this oil as a facial cleanser or moisturizer. Add several drops of this oil to your preferred cream. The oil works by preventing the bacteria from thriving on your skin. This can also help in balancing the system's production of sebum. When regularly used, the oil is effective in preventing scars from developing after your face has been cleared of acne.

8. Earache. Warm the bottle of the oil and after two minutes, massage a few drops of the oil on the skin that surrounds the ears and along the throat.

9. Headache. Gently massage a few drops of this oil on your temples and at the nape of the neck to relieve yourself from the pain.

10. Menstrual cramps. Massage several drops of the oil on your lower abdomen and apply a hot compress until the pain is relieved.

## Unwinding Using the Scent of Lavender

Lavender oil has healing effects. When you are not bothered with certain health issues, you will have an easier time sleeping. If you are losing sleep because of the following health problems, do not hesitate and use this oil to begin sleeping soundly every night.

### 1. Dandruff

There are some people who aren't comfortable when they have flakes in the scalp, even when it is time to sleep. Aside from the itch, the flakes get scattered all over the pillows and beddings. Do this regimen for several days or until all the flakes are gone in order to get rid of dandruff. Wet your hair with warm water and towel it to dry. Put 15 drops of lavender oil in a container and mix this with two tablespoons of almond or olive oil. Heat the mixture in the microwave until it reaches the warmth that will feel comfortable on your scalp. Massage the oil onto your scalp. Wrap your head with a warm towel, wait for an hour before you shampoo and rinse your hair.

## 2. Itchy skin

Lavender essential oil has natural anti-inflammatory properties. There are many causes of itchy skin, such as insect bites, allergies and skin problems. The oil can help reduce the itch, swelling and redness. You simply need to drop the oil on the affected area. Wait for 15 minutes until the skin has absorbed the oil. You can add one more drop if the itch is severe. If this is the first time that you are going to do this, make sure that you first wait how your skin will react to the oil. If it becomes itchier, this means that you are allergic to the oil, so stop using it. If not, repeat the process after six hours and continue doing so until the itch is totally gone.

If the itch is caused by eczema, which typically happens to kids, add several drops of the oil to a carrier oil or your child's favorite lotion. Shake the mixture and gently massage this on the affected area. This can give your child instant comfort. This will make it easier for him/her to sleep.

3. Stress and anxiety

There are many causes of stress, but no matter what your problems are, you should not let any of these affect the quality of your sleep. When you are troubled and you are also finding it hard to sleep, you will have a harder time in dealing with your worries. You have to get your mind clear and your body refreshed in order to face your problems and do whatever's necessary to solve these. You can only do that if you have rested completely and your body was able to recharge.

Lavender oil helps you relax. The scent makes you feel drowsy. It is best that you develop a nightly regimen of using the oil on your warm bath before you go to bed and diffuse it to keep you company as you sleep through the night. The smell of this oil helps in lowering your heart rate and blood pressure, the two factors that surge when you are constantly faced with problems and stressful factors. You can diffuse the oil and put the container on your nightstand. You can also use dried herbs instead of the oil. Put the pieces in a container and place it near your bed.

While the scent of lavender can help you relax and sleep easier, you have to help yourself by doing the right activities and habits. For one, make sure that you lessen your caffeine and alcohol consumption. Help yourself by fixing your room in such a way that it looks tempting to sleep. Do not bring your work at home, especially if it is causing you stress.

## 4. Fatigue

There are certain people who easily fall asleep when they are too tired. There are some who find it difficult to sleep in this condition, especially when they can feel that parts of their body are aching. Before you sleep, relax the part of your body that is aching with the help of this essential oil. For example, if you have aching feet, prepare a hot foot bath and add five drops of lavender oil. Linger as you soak your feet and try to relax. There are many pores in the soles of the feet, which enable the oil to enter your bloodstream. Through this, you will feel the soothing effects and after several minutes, you will no longer feel the pain.

If your whole body is aching, a 10-minute warm bath, with a few drops of this oil mixed with water, is your best bet. For other aches, you can gently massage the affected parts with this oil and feel instant relief and calmness.

5. Fever

Children and even adults often find it hard to sleep when they are running a fever, especially when the temperature is quite high. If you can't bring the patient immediately to the hospital to seek medical attention or you still want to observe if the condition will improve, use this oil because it will help in lowering the temperature and in relieving the patient from the aches and discomfort that he/he feels.

It is a common practice to sponge the body of kids and babies with tepid water when they have a fever. This will work faster and more effective if you are going to add a drop of the oil into the water. Do the process gently and have a dry towel ready. Make sure that the patient does not get chilled because this can make matters worse. You can also perform the same process to adults.

The process is done along with the proper medications for fever. The medicines will also help in cooling off the body by releasing the heat that is causing the high temperatures. You will sponge the patient's body as you wait for the medicines to take effect.

6. Insomnia

This kind of sickness is commonly treated with medications. If the latter fails to work and you are still having a hard time falling into sleep at night, you should try using lavender oil. You can place the oil in a diffuser and allow the smell spread across your room. You can also massage the oil on your wrists and temple, or apply some on your pillow. For many elderly people who are insomniac, this process works better than taking medications.

Babies and young kids are also prone to have difficulties in sleeping at night. The reason for this is that they typically sleep most of the time during the day. You can allow this phase to pass and wait until they develop normal sleeping habits. If it is taking too long though, and many people in your house are having trouble sleeping at night because of a loud baby, then you have to do something about it. Calm your baby's nerves and help them relax before you put them to bed. Add a drop of lavender oil with carrier oil and gently massage it on your baby's body. You can also add two drops of lavender oil in your baby's bedtime bath.

7. Jet lag

If travel is an important part of your job, you have to learn how to deal with jet lag and make sure that it doesn't cause you quality sleep. Bring this oil with you wherever you go. While traveling, dab some oil on your wrists and temples. This will help you relax and clear your head while you are on your way to your destination. You can combine lavender with other essential oils to get faster and better effects. You can use oils such as clary sage, Neroli, frankincense and rosemary.

You have to help your body adjust to the different time zones of the places that you will visit. This way, you can maximize the time that you will spend at each destination without getting sick or bothered due to lack of sleep.

Using lavender oil is not exclusive to those who are sick or have difficulty falling and staying asleep. You can make this part of your nightly habit to ensure a sound sleep every night.

# Chapter 3

## Vetiver Essential Oil

Vetiver essential oil (Vetiveria zizanioides) has a rich and earthy smell. This is a popular oil that is used to obtain better sleep, but it takes time before you get used to its aroma. For starters, you can mix this oil with oils that have lighter scents, including lavender. Little by little, take away the other oil until you get immune in using vetiver on its own.

The oil is extracted from the roots of the plants through the process of steam distillation. Although this is not as widely known as the most common essential oils, the benefits and uses of vetiver date back in ancient history. It has an exotic scent that you have to learn to appreciate in order to benefit from its effects.

Make sure that you only get the best quality of this oil. It has many positive properties, which include calming effects, antispasmodic, antiseptic, warming, stimulates the circulatory system, gives sedative effects to the nervous system and a lot more. This is mainly promoted to help people get better sleep, especially at times when you are unable to relax and you feel very restless. It guides you towards a peaceful sleep and sometimes gives you crazy dreams.

This oil also affects your emotions and inner longings. Its aroma can affect what you are really feeling inside. This can help you get more motivated to obtain your passion and overcome all the hurdles that you are faced with. This can help you understand your core, which is something that certain people fear. If you are not yet ready to accept who you really are, you may want to stay away from this oil until the time that you have lost such fear.

When choosing the vetiver essential oil with superior quality, you have to consider several guidelines. The variety of plants where the oil is obtained is grown from the indigenous regions across the globe. The harvest season is done when the temperature is right in order to preserve the molecules of the oil.

Everything goes through the process of testing before it is packed and made available in the market.

In using this oil, make sure that you perform a skin patch test when you are a first time user. Never use this more often than what's required because this can lead to skin sensitization. Avoid its direct contact with your nose, ears and eyes. Pregnant women and children must seek approval and guidance before using this kind of essential oil.

Various Uses of Vetiver Oil

Aside from being an effective tool to put you to sleep, this oil is also used to deal with the following health concerns:

1. Anxiety. It gives you a grounding feeling when you are having anxiety attacks. You can diffuse the oil and inhale the scent. You can also massage this over your solar plexus or at the center of the chest area, where your heart is located, until you are feeling better.

2. Skin care. You can make this a part of your beauty regimen and let it deal with various skin problems, such as acne, aging, oily and irritated skin. You can

mix a drop of vetiver oil with six drops of coconut oil. Massage the mixture on your skin before you go to bed. You can also mix the oil with an anti-aging cream of your choice to boost its effectiveness. The antiseptic properties of the oil work in cleansing your skin against the bacteria and dirt that cause acne breakout. Wash your face before you apply a mixture of a drop of this oil and three drops of coconut oil.

4. Arthritis. You can mix several drops of this oil to your preferred pain-relieving lotion and massage it over the affected areas of your body.

5. Balance. This works great for people who have problems in balancing their weight and as a result, they often fall down or topple over. With its grounding effects, you can solve your dilemma by making this part of your daily regimen. It is enough to inhale its scent. You can choose to diffuse it or pour some drops on your shirt or handkerchief. When you stroll, run or jog, it is recommended that you massage this oil first at the reflex points of your feet.

6. ADD/ADHD. If you have loved ones who are suffering from this kind of disease, you will appreciate the calming effects that the vetiver oil can provide. This will help the person with the disability to calm down, especially when it's time to sleep and rest. This way, the other members of the family can also rest without getting troubled with sudden outbursts of tantrums and emotions. You can massage the oil on the feet and toes or put several drops into the warm bath of the person with ADD/ADHD. You can also pour a few drops into their pillows and beddings to help them sleep through the night.

7. Dandruff. To deal with this problem, mix two drops of this oil with two drops of lavender oil and six drops of coconut oil. Before you sleep, massage this onto your scalp. You can wrap your head with a soft cloth so that the oil won't scatter on your pillow as you doze off. Rinse your hair in the morning. Repeat the regimen until you have gotten rid of the flakes.

8. Trauma. No matter what has caused the trauma, this oil can help the person feel calm and grounded.

You can opt to diffuse this and let the patient inhale the scent. This will have an instant calming effect, which will lessen the fear and help the person face whatever has caused the problem. In this case, the better way to use this oil is through topical application. You can massage the oil over the heart and solar plexus of the individual, and gently go over the back of the neck in order to release the tension.

9. Anorexia. If you have this kind of problem, do not wait until it becomes severe before you do something about it. Aside from medications, use this oil as part of your regimen in order to deal with this health condition. Massage the oil over your abdomen and chest. You can also diffuse the oil and inhale it whenever you are in the room. Through time, the oil will help in balancing your emotional state, which has led you to have eating disorders and end up with this sickness. As you follow the process, never miss out on the medications that your doctor has given you.

10. Depression. The oil helps a person achieve a healthier emotional state. It unlocks whatever it is that you are keeping inside and help you deal with it.

It promotes balance of your nervous system and hormones. You can use this aromatically or you can also use this in massaging your body. If the condition is severe, make sure that you seek the doctor's help to give you proper medications. This way, the oil will perform better in aiding the medicines to help you in dealing with the problem.

How to Use Vetiver Oil to Sleep Better

There are various conditions that hinder a person's ability to get sufficient rest. This oil can help you deal with the following:

1. Insomnia. When using this oil topically, make sure that you only use a little. Putting too much of this oil can make you feel tired upon waking up in the morning. You can gently massage a few drops of this oil at the back of your neck or at the soles of your feet. It will instantly make you feel calm and grounded.

2. Nightmares. There are some people who often experience nightmares, which is the reason why they have trouble sleeping. They are already anticipating

the nightly terrors. Try diffusing this essential oil, so that it can accompany you as you sleep. This will help you sleep peacefully and wake up in the morning feeling refreshed. You can also spray some on your beddings or pillows.

Vetiver oil also works wonders for children who are only beginning to get accustomed to a normal sleeping pattern. Its scent will help your child to feel sleepy when it's time to go to bed and stay peacefully asleep until it is time to wake up.

If you intend to apply the oil topically on your child, always dilute it first. Avoid applying the oil anywhere near their eyes. For kids who are 9 years old and below, you can dilute a drop of this oil in a teaspoon of vegetable oil. Gently apply this at the soles of the feet of the child. You can put an additional drop of vetiver oil for kids who are 10 years and above.

Most adults can use this oil as it is. If you are uncertain whether or not you are sensitive to this, it is safer to dilute it first and perform a skin patch test.

# Chapter 4

# Roman Chamomile Essential Oil

When it comes to the best oils that are used to help people sleep better, Roman Chamomile essential oil or Chammaemelum nobile, is always included at the top of the list. This is known for its relaxing and soothing scent. It has a light floral scent that you will instantly love.

This oil has been used in ancient history. During times of a war, the ancient Romans believed that this oil can be used to boost the courage and clear the minds of people. This is also beneficial to other plants; hence, it was given the moniker as plant's physician. The scent is absorbed by nearby plants, and benefit in the process.

The unique properties of this oil include anti-inflammatory, anti-infectious, anti-parasitic, and, of course, it is calming and relaxing. Aside from essential oils, chamomile is also widely used as a tea flavor, which is favored by those who have a hard time sleeping at night.

This can also help heal a person in a spiritual level. You can use its aroma when meditating, especially at times when you feel down and discouraged. This will remind you of your purpose and the scent will help you understand what your core is trying to say. If you are feeling helpless and hopeless, you will have a clearer understanding of what led to this and what are your options to get out of this state. This has the effect of making your ego softer, so that you can think clearly and decide on things objectively.

This can also help people who are experiencing anxiety. This will help you find inner peace in all areas of your life.

Aside from helping you doze off without any hassles, this essential oil can help in healing the following health problems.

1. Detoxification. Massage the oil on the reflex points of the feet or in the area where the liver is located. This will help the liver to function at its best in order

to help your system get rid of unhealthy and harmful toxins.

2. Wounds and cuts. The oil has healing properties that can reduce inflammation. You can dilute the oil and use this to massage over the affected parts, add several drops to hot/cold compress or add the oil into your bath water. Soak for at least 10 minutes and this will give you an instant feeling of relief and you will notice that the wounds will begin to heal. The complete healing process will take several days or weeks to heal, depending on its condition.

3. Depression. You must never disregard the feeling of depression. You never know what your mind is capable of thinking when you are quite down. You can deal with your problems better if you have a clear mind and if you are feeling lighter. To get to this state, make it part of your regimen before going to bed at night to diffuse this oil and inhale this as you go to sleep. You can also apply a few drops to your pillows and beddings.

4. Allergies. If you have seasonal allergies, make sure that you are equipped with this oil before the season

begins. Always diffuse this inside your home in ways that you can often smell the scent. When your allergies flare up, massage a few drops of the oil at the soles of your feet.

5. Menopause. When you are entering this stage, your body undergoes a lot of changes that it often leads you to become more irritable. Massaging the oil at the back of your neck and on your feet will help in calming your endocrine system. Follow this regimen every night before you go to bed until you are feeling okay and you have gotten used to the changes that this stage brings about.

6. Muscle aches and tension. You can use the combination of Roman chamomile and coconut oil to massage the affected area. Make sure that you go over gently, especially when the pain is unbearable. Repeat the process until the pain is completely gone.

You can use Roman chamomile essential oil in massaging your legs and feet if this area of your body feels restless. The oil will have a soothing effect on your muscles and calm down your nervous system. In effect, your feet will feel more relaxed.

7. Irritated skin. This feels itchy and can lead to rashes if you can't stop the itch. You can soothe the skin by adding three drops of this oil to a teaspoon of carrier oil. Massage the mixture to the affected area in a gentle manner. Refrain from scratching the itch as much as possible. Children may find it very hard to stop scratching the affected area. You have to explain the process and tell the kids to wait for a magic to happen or when the itch will fade with the wonders of the oil.

8. Parasites. There are Roman chamomile oils that you can take internally. You can pour the oil into empty veggie capsules or add some drops to a tea, and give this to the person who has parasites. If you aren't used in taking the oil orally, you can opt to massage it in the abdominal area or at the reflex points of your feet.

9. Bee sting. Instead of feeling the pain, use the oil to get instant relief and to get rid of the swelling. You can use this neat if you are certain that you are not allergic to it, by dropping a tiny amount of oil to the affected area. You can also dilute this with coconut oil

and use the mixture to gently massage the part where you were stung.

10.  Skin problems. You can add a small amount of this oil to your preferred beauty product or coconut oil. Apply the mixture like how you would a regular beauty product on the problem areas. This can help in healing skin problems, which include eczema, boils, acne, dermatitis and dryness.

11. Sciatica. Massage the oil on your lower back and hips, to the aching legs and the reflex points of the hands and feet. The process will give relief to the sciatic nerve, while the scent makes you feel lighter and calm.

12. Fear. There are times when you suddenly feel fearful of something that you don't really understand. You may also get shocked over petty things, which can make you feel emotionally unstable. This is the best time to inhale the scent of Roman chamomile essential oil. It will instantly give you a sense of balance and calmness.

# How to Use Roman Chamomile to Help You Sleep Better

There are certain conditions that make it harder for a person to sleep or remain asleep. This essential oil can help in attending to the following conditions:

1. Children who find it hard to sleep. When you are a parent to kids who can't sleep peacefully at night, it follows that you will also lose precious sleep. Children and infants will benefit from the aroma of this oil. You can gently massage the oil to their feet, but make sure that you have diluted it first. The oil can help your kids sleep through the night. This can also help in healing certain problems that make it harder for kids to sleep, including fever, toothache, earache, stomach ache and other kinds of pains.

2. Hyperactivity. If a person finds it hard to sleep due to this reason, you can diffuse the oil and allow the person to inhale its scent. This will give him/her instant calmness. You can also massage the oil to the soles of the feet and make this a nightly habit.

3. Irritability. No matter what has caused this emotion, you will find it hard to sleep if the reason why you are feeling this way keeps on bugging you. You need to feel inner peace and calm your nerves. You can massage the oil at the back of your neck until you feel lighter and sleepy. You can also inhale its scent and apply a few drops on your pillow and beddings.

4. Insomnia. A lot of people who have this condition try to fight it off by drinking chamomile tea when it is already bed time. To make the tea more potent, you can add one drop of chamomile essential oil to your cup. You can also apply the oil topically by gently massaging this on your feet and back.

5. Fatigue. While there are some people who easily doze off when they are pretty tired, there are also those who feel the pain and have a hard time falling into a peaceful sleep. Ask someone to perform a full body massage using this oil. In the end, apply a few drops at the base of your head.

There are various ways to use this oil to help you have a better and more peaceful sleep. Here are some useful techniques that you may want to try.

- When washing your hair, you can add a drop of this oil to your shampoo. The scent will cling to your hair and you will feel its effects throughout the day. You can also combine this with your lotion or moisturizer. Aside from the aroma, the oil helps in making your hair and skin retain the youthful appeal.
- Aside from chamomile tea, you can also add a drop of this oil to your chosen hot drinks at night. This will help your nerves to calm and prepare your mind that it is about to doze off.
- You can combine this with lavender and massage your body with the mixture before you go to bed. The effect is soothing and very relaxing.
- This is also a useful tool to people who need to stay awake late at night and want to fall asleep fast the moment they hit the bed. In this case, you can diffuse the oil or use this to massage the reflex points of your hands and feet.

# Chapter 5

## Ylang Ylang Essential Oil

Ylang ylang essential oil (Cananga odorata) has an overwhelming floral and sweet scent. It is interesting to note that the wild flower where it originated in ancient times had no scent. Its nice smell is favored as a room deodorizer, but aside from the aroma, it has a lot of healing properties as well.

Ylang ylang essential oil is sedative, tonic, antiseptic, antispasmodic and antidepressant. The oil benefits a person's endocrine, hormonal and cardiovascular system, especially the heart. This helps a person connect to his/her emotions and spirituality. This allows you to hear out your inner child. Through this, you will discover what really makes you happy and contented.

Aside from helping you sleep better at night, the oil has other health benefits and can bring positive effects to certain health problems, which include the following:

1. Hair Loss. Mix a drop of this oil with several drops of coconut oil. Massage this onto your scalp before you sleep at night. You can wrap your head with a soft cloth so that the oil won't scatter on your pillow.

2. Diabetes. You will find it easier to deal with the condition when you massage the oil to the reflex points of your feet and on the area where your pancreas are located. Perform this nightly to help your body attain balance.

3. Emotional dilemma. If you have heart problems, like getting your heart broken, you are very much in love or you feel unloved, make it a habit to put a drop of this oil in the area where your heart is. This is best done before you meditate. This will help you in accepting the emotions and removing any kinds of negativity.

4. Low sex drive. To boost your sex drive, you can diffuse the oil in the bedroom. You can also massage this to your shoulders and feet. It can also help to inhale the scent directly from an open bottle at least once a day.

5. High blood pressure. The oil has a calming effect on your nervous system. You simply have to massage the oil to the reflex points of your feet and hands. You can also massage this directly on the area where your heart is.

How to Use Ylang Ylang Oil to Help You Sleep Better

There are certain conditions that affect the quality of sleep. You can use the ylang ylang essential oil in addressing the following concerns:

1. Conflicting emotions. There are days when you can't sleep because of the emotional turmoil that you are going through. In many cases, you can diffuse the scent into the room and you will feel better as you inhale it. If you are angry, put a drop in your palm and put it over your nose to smell. When you are feeling restless, you can inhale from the bottle or put a drop of the oil to your lotion and massage this on your hands and feet. Massage the oil on the area near your heart if you are fearful, even when you aren't sure what the cause is.

2. Colic. When your baby has colic, you have to help him/her calm down and stop crying. Diffusing the oil will do wonders, but to see the results faster, dilute a drop of this oil to a teaspoon of carrier oil and massage this to the feet of your baby.

3. Fatigue. If this is causing you to lose sleep, massage two drops of the oil to the soles of your feet. Allow the process to take effect while you breathe deeply. After a while, your body will relax and you will find it easier to doze off.

4. Insomnia. If this is the cause why you are losing sleep, massage two drops of this oil onto your nape or at the soles of your feet.

You can try this recipe to help you sleep better. Mix two drops of ylang ylang and three drops of French lavender. Add the mixture to your warm bath and soak your body for at least 10 minutes. Close your eyes, try to relax as you inhale the oil's scent.

You can also experiment with another recipe using this oil along with other essential oils. You will create a mixture that you will use for a whole body massage.

Perform the task before you go to bed. The recipe includes two drops of ylang ylang oil, two drops each of oils that include tangerine, orange, lavender, marjoram and chamomile and an ounce of carrier oil.

# Chapter 6

## Bergamot Essential Oil

Bergamot essential oil (Citrus bergamia) comes from the peel of an exotic fruit. It has a citrus and sweet smell. The aroma has a certain depth that will make you feel calm and relaxed. The effect that this oil has is different from other citrus oils, which tend to stimulate one's mood. The scent of bergamot is bright, but also relaxing at the same time.

Its healing properties include anti-inflammatory, antiseptic, uplifting, digestive, sedative, analgesic, antibacterial, neuro-protective and antispasmodic. It is used to address physical health concerns, but works best in promoting emotional wellness. It also helps boost a person's acceptance of who he/she really is, self-worth and love. It also makes it easier for you to accept your flaws and love yourself despite that. When used regularly in meditation, the aroma of this oil can help you face your fears.

Its properties make it a good antidepressant oil. The scent will make it easier for you to process your pain, fear, rejections and shame. This also works for those who are suffering from addiction and certain compulsions. It helps bring joy when you are clouded by sadness and confidence when shyness seems too empowering.

Here's a list of the health conditions where you can use bergamot essential oil.

1. Addiction. No matter what it is that you are addicted to, you can use this oil to overcome the problem. Make sure that you always smell its scent throughout the day. Diffuse it in your room and apply a drop on the collar of your shirt. At night before you sleep, massage your feet with a drop of this oil. It is also important to apply a drop of this oil on your solar plexus two times a day.

Perform the regimen using the oil in conjunction with the medications and exercises that your doctor advised you to follow. This way, the road to recovery becomes faster.

2. Loss of appetite. This can happen as a result of a sickness, lack of the will to eat, depression and many more. If it is taking a long time and your health is already suffering, do not wait any longer before you do something about it. If you will allow this to continue, you may develop other illnesses and your body will lose its needed energy. To deal with the problem, apply a drop or two of this oil on your stomach and gently massage it. Perform this several times within the day and continue until you have regained your appetite.

3. Cold sores. When you see a sign of a cold sore, do not wait until it fully develops. Apply a tiny amount on the affected area and repeat the process until the sore is gone. You can also dilute this with coconut oil and apply to the affected area thrice a day or more often if necessary.

5. Brain injury. This can happen as a result of an accident or as an effect of an existing sickness. To relieve yourself from the pain and other effects of the condition, you can directly inhale the scent of the oil from its bottle. Follow the practice several times a

day. You can also put a drop of the oil on the back of the neck, and then massage it gently while you inhale the scent.

6. Skin problems. If your skin is oily, you can use this oil as an astringent. Apply a drop to a cotton ball and clean your face with it. If you have pimples and acne, you can dab a tiny amount of oil at the affected part and wait for the skin to absorb it. In both cases, make sure that you avoid getting exposed to direct sunlight. Perform a skin patch test first and proceed only when you are certain that you are not allergic to this oil.

7. Indigestion. To deal with this, apply two drops of oil to your stomach and massage it gently. Perform this each time before you eat or until you are already feeling fine.

8. Infection. Clean the affected area with water and allow it to dry. Put two drops around the affected area and wait until the oil seeps through the skin. It will also help to inhale the oil directly from the bottle several times within the day.

9. Intestinal worms. The condition is usually not painful. It can be hard to detect if you have these worms inside of you. There are signs that may point out to this reason. In this case, use two drops of bergamot oil. Apply the oil to your abdomen and massage it gently. Perform this several times a day.

10. Rheumatoid Arthritis. You can use two drops of oil to massage over the painful area of your body twice a day.

11. Urinary Tract Infection. Aside from proper medications, the recovery process is faster to those who use this oil to deal with the condition. You can add several drops of oil to the water that you drink. You can also opt to massage the oil at the area of your body where the kidneys, urethra and bladder are located. Perform the massage several times a day.

Self-Healing with the Use of Bergamot Oil

There are so many emotions and issues that this oil helps to address. If you are constantly faced with a lot of emotional turmoil, never forget to have a bottle of this oil handy. The oil works wonders for the following emotional dilemmas:

1. Agitation. When you are agitated, it is hard to focus and you will also find it difficult to sleep. Put a drop of the oil on your palm, rub your hands together and put these over your nose. Savor the smell for a minute, or longer if necessary.

2. Lack of confidence. There are times when you can't help but feel shy. This happens as a result of a traumatic experience or by simply feeling like you are hit with a lot of butterflies in your stomach. During an important day, like when you have a presentation or a job interview, exude confidence by inhaling the scent of this oil at the start of the day. You can also put a drop of bergamot oil on your abdomen and massage it gently several times a day.

3. Stress. There are many kinds of stress that this oil can help you deal with and overcome. When you are suffering from mental stress due to information or work overload, you can inhale its scent directly from the bottle as often as necessary. Rubbing your abdomen with a drop of bergamot oil will also help in

this case. If the stress is caused by your performance and how you want many things to get done at once, diffuse the oil and try to pause and breathe deeply several times a day. You can also opt to use the oil in giving your feet a quick massage in the midst of a hectic schedule. If you are dealing with environmental stress, simply open the bottle of the oil and savor its smell as often as needed.

How to Use Bergamot Essential Oil to Help You Sleep Better

With so many uses, it is a bonus that this oil is also effective in promoting a sound and quality sleep. Here are some of the ways to get this done:

1. Add 10 drops of the oil to your warm bath. Soak in the water for at least 10 minutes. This will allow the oil to penetrate your skin, while you inhale its scent in the process. This will make you feel calm and ready to doze off after you are done rinsing.

2. Have a whole body massage before going to bed. Add two drops of this oil top an unscented lotion and massage it gently all over your body.

3. Diffuse the oil and let the aroma linger in the room as you doze off.

# Chapter 7:

## Sandalwood Essential Oil

Sandalwood essential oil (Santalum album) has an earthy and woody aroma. It comes from the wood of the sandalwood tree and the oils are extracted through the process of steam distillation. Its scent is rich but not overpowering.

It is known for its many healing properties, such as antiseptic, sedative, antidepressant, astringent, aphrodisiac, tonic and antitumor. This is mostly used in pampering the skin and in dealing with health issues in the nervous system and bones. It is believed to help in relieving pain caused by brain disease and in making the condition better.

Sandalwood is widely used in meditation. This is a 'spiritual' oil – the kind that helps a person to achieve a peaceful state and let go of his/her worries. The oil has various uses and is believed to benefit those who are suffering from the following health problems:

1. Alzheimer's. The oil has the capacity to improve the condition of the patient. You simply have to massage three drops of the oil to the nape several times a day. Move gently and allow the person smell the aroma as you go about the massage.

2. Bronchitis. Aside from taking proper medications, the use of this oil can help in alleviating the symptoms and in helping you to heal faster. Massage two drops of oil on your throat and over the chest three times a day.

3. Comatose. A person who is in a coma may still be capable of feeling. To help him/her heal faster, apply two drops of sandalwood oil to the back of the neck and forehead and massage these parts gently. Perform the massage several times a day.

4. Hemorrhoids. A drop of the oil on the affected area can help relieve the pain and inflammation. You can do this as often as needed.

5. Dry hair. Mix several drops of this oil with coconut oil. Use it to massage your scalp. Let the oil sit in your

hair for an hour. Rinse it all off and towel your hair dry.

How to Use Sandalwood Essential Oil to Help You Sleep Better

This oil can deal with the following conditions that are affecting the quality of your sleep:

1. Back pain. Before you lay and try to doze up, ask someone to massage your back. Use three drops of this oil in the process. You can also mix it with other oils, like wintergreen, to make the effect more potent.

2. Insomnia. Your goal is to command your brain to stop thinking so that you can sleep without any hassles. To get this done, massage two drops of this oil over your brow. Breathe in the scent as you perform the massage.

3. Stress. The best way to deal with it is by diffusing the oil. Breathe deeply and allow your nerves to relax as your mind let go of the worries and the causes of such emotion.

This oil is used in a lot of ways to help you sleep peacefully at night. This is best utilized through diffusion and topical application. It is not recommended to take sandalwood essential oil orally because this may have toxic effects. If you want to try taking this internally, ask a medical professional about it first and bring samples of the brand of oil that you wish to consume.

The oil has relaxing and calming effects, but to make it more potent, you can mix this with carrier oils, such as sweet almond, jojoba and avocado.

# Conclusion

Thank you again for purchasing this book!

I hope this book was able to help you to understand what kinds of essential oils can help you sleep soundly and peacefully every night. Aside from this kind of benefit, this book hopes to enlighten you about the other uses of the oils and how to apply the oils to experience the positive effects.

The next step is to head to the nearest store, find the right scents and start incorporating the use of essential oils into your daily life.

Finally, if you got any value out of this book, then I'd like to ask you for a favor, would you be kind enough to leave a review for this book on Amazon? It'd be greatly appreciated!


Thank you and good luck!